Dr. med. Andreas Ganz
Bernhard Johannes Schmidt

AF198951

PLAINTEXT compact

The ASPERGER Syndrome

for Physicians

Dr. med. Andreas Ganz
Bernhard J. Schmidt

PLAINTEXT compact
**The ASPERGER Syndrome
for Physicians**

© 2019 Bernhard J. Schmidt,
Oberwarmensteinach, Germany
All Rights reserved.

ISBN: 978-3749469833

translated from
KLARTEXT kompakt
Das ASPERGER Syndrom für Ärzte
© 2016 Bernhard J. Schmidt,
ISBN: 9783739240893

Production and Publishing:
BoD – Books on Demand, Norderstedt, Germany

Bibliographic information of the German National Library:
The German National Library lists this publication
in the German National Bibliography; detailed bibliographic
Data are available online at http://dnb.dnb.de.

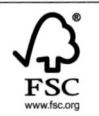

Table of content

I. PREFACE

When reading the book title many doctors spontaneously go through the thought: "This is none of my business, I have no autistic people in practice."
This is exactly where a great deal of the health care problem for people in the autistic spectrum already lies. With a prevalence of approximately 0.5 percent, at least this percentage of autistic individuals should be represented in every practice. If one also takes into account the greatly increased risk of illness, the proportion of patients would actually have to be around one to two percent - depending on the specialization. Over the past few years, studies have repeatedly shown a significantly reduced "health-related quality of life" in autistic individuals. How serious the health problems of people from the autistic spectrum are, shows a very large and current study:

„Results: During the observed period, 24 358 (0.91%) individuals in the general population died, whereas the corresponding figure for individuals with ASD was 706 (2.60%; OR = 2.56; 95% CI 2.38–2.76). Cause-specific analyses showed elevated mortality in ASD for almost all analysed diagnostic categories. Mortality and patterns

for cause-specific mortality were partly moderated by gender and general intellectual ability.

Conclusions:

Premature mortality was markedly increased in ASD owing to a multitude of medical conditions. "

[Premature mortality in autism spectrum disorder; Tatja Hirvikoski, Ellenor Mittendorfer-Rutz, Marcus Boman, Henrik Larsson, Paul Lichtenstein, Sven Bölte; The British Journal of Psychiatry Nov 2015, DOI: 10.1192/bjp.bp.114.160192]

And so comes Prof. Dr. med. Bölte in the "British Journal of Psychiatry" concludes:

"We were able to show that people with autism spectrum disorder (ASD) have a higher mortality risk for almost all causes of death, **which is why all medical disciplines need knowledge about autism** *"*

Quotes after: http://psylex.de/entwicklung/autismus/sterblichkeit.html

With a steadily increasing prevalence and of course at the same time, the number of diagnosed autists needs urgent improvement of their medical care. The goal should be that there are nationwide and depending on the respective population corresponding specialized general medical practices.

These can then serve both as a first port of call for autistics and as an intermediary to appropriate medical specialists with accompanying information about the special needs of the autistic patient.

In dental practices, at least anxiety patients are already being given special attention.

But unfortunately, only dental anxiety with the resulting consequences is perceived so far:

„Dentists face daily dental fears of varying intensity. However, according to a study on the prevalence of dental phobia in standard German dental practices, only 0.5% met the criteria for phobia. The dentist often meets only in emergency on such patients. Then there is already an urgent need for treatment, a gentle painless treatment is not always possible and so these emergency visits are often a further confirmation in the vicious circle of fear."

[Lenk M, Berth H, Joraschky P, Petrowski K, Weidner K, Hannig C: Fear of dental treatment—an underrecognized symptom in people with impaired mental health. Dtsch Arztebl Int 2013; 110(31–32): 517–22. DOI: 10.3238/arztebl.2013.0517]

But the problems that prevent a doctor's visit are much more far-reaching and complex with autistic people.

For autistics, anxiety and stress are key issues - but they are not just another group of anxiety patients! The fear is not limited to the treatment.

Fear and stress prevent autistic people not only from visiting a dentist, but from a doctor, no matter what specialty. On the other hand, anxiety and stress are also the cause of many diseases, as shown by the diathesis stress model. This can be helpful in both the history and diagnosis as well as the treatment.

As in the other volumes of the series *"Plaintext compact. The Asperger Syndrome"*, so here too is largely dispensed with the indication of sources and studies. The underlying explanations with the scientific basis can be found in the books from the series *"Bernhard J. Schmidt: Autistic and Society. An angry change of perspective"*.

Even if the male form is used consistently in this book, the autistic girls and women should not be overlooked. Already the necessary check-ups are a big hurdle for many autistic women!

Thus, physicians in private practice in all disciplines should be confronted with, or work towards, autistics in equal numbers.

II. THEORY

Although the diagnostic criteria of autism as "impairment of social interaction and communication" include the interaction between at least two persons, autism has so far only been considered isolated and intrapersonally and by means of cognitive psychology.

On the other hand, the approach presented here is based on an interpersonal, socio-psychological perspective.

Anxiety and stress cause somatic as well as psychological problems / illnesses and at the same time prevent the treatment!

There are two areas that are responsible for the development of anxiety and stress as opposed to neurologically typical people (NT people). On the one hand, there is a marked difference in communication and, on the other, in sensory perception.

1   Communication

Since the 1950s, social psychology has shown that most NT people communicate with each other unconsciously and non-verbally. This communication works through facial expressions, gestures, the imitation of the posture, movement and voice tune of the opposite, through synchronization ...

The carrier medium for unconscious group communication and social "grooming" is gossip, which makes up about 70% of NT people's communication. This unconscious group communication serves both the automatic orientation, so as "autopilot", as well as energy-saving mode. At the same time, unconscious group communication establishes belonging to the own group and distinguishing it from outside groups. These group processes serve to a not inconsiderable extent also the avoidance of fear and / or the dismantling of fear.

1.1 Absence of unconscious group communication

Autistic people lack this unconscious group communication. This means that autistics can neither imitate their counterparts nor interpret facial expressions or gestures.

It also means that autistic communication differs significantly from NT people because gossip is dropped and pure factual information is communicated. As a result, autistics often appear to be very silent - but also unfriendly, because the communicative "grooming" is omitted.

As a result, the speech melody of autistic individuals is often monotone and body movements appear wooden. For autistics this means

1.) No autopilot, that is, that autistic people can not unconsciously orient themselves to the behavior of the group. Autists have to orient and structure themselves always and actively.

2.) No unconscious group affiliation and thus no participation in the fear-avoidance behavior of and anxiety reduction by groups.

3.) No energy-saving mode, but an energy-consuming active coping with the tasks and challenges of the environment.

4.) In addition, the behavior of others often appears irrational, unpredictable and frightening.

5.) Autistic people often suffer exclusion, marginalization and bullying due to the lack of unconscious group communication.

Already all these points lead to high levels of anxiety and stress in autistics, as several studies have shown.
However, there are also the sensory features of autistic people.

2   Sensory features

In the brevity of the presentation is a simplifying distinction between a sensory hypersensitivity and hypo-sensitivity. This is a hypersensitivity especially in the field of the senses, ie, see, hear, smell and sense of touch. Hyposensitivity, however, in proprioception.

2.1   Hypersensitive exteroception

For the development of stress but also of phobias, the hypersensitive perception is largely responsible. This is mainly due to a filter weakness, which means that irrelevant or disturbing stimuli are not automatically filtered out. Thus, environmental stimuli that NT people do not perceive are not only perceived by autistics, but often even as painful or irritating.

On the one hand, this hypersensitivity refers to acoustic stimuli that are perceived by autistic people as if NT people were equipped with a too loud hearing aid. And as with hearing aids, it is difficult to filter out acoustic signals (for example, a conversation partner against background noise = party filter). Noise, such as the ticking of a clock, often unnoticed by NT people, can be perceived by the autistic as very distracting and irritating.

Particularly in the area of the doctor's office, the hypersensitive olfactory perception of autistic people is of central importance. This begins in the waiting room with the partly unpleasant odors of the other patients and goes on to the odors of disinfectants, etc., with which autistics are confronted in practices.

When it comes to sight, it is mainly to bright light and flickering lamps that are very disturbing to painful for autistic people.

But attention to touch sensitivity, which makes touch often uncomfortable to painful, is also important in treating autistic individuals.

2.2   Hyposensitive proprioception

Although not important for the development of anxiety and stress, but important for the diagnosis, is the often described hyposensitivity of proprioception. Thus, heat and cold are not adequately perceived by autistics and pain sensations are also often absent, e.g. with dental problems. As a result, the self-perception and pain perception of autistics is unfortunately rather unreliable for the diagnosis. So if an autist has no pain, it does not mean that there is no disease / injury.

3 Diathesis stress model

Unfortunately, autism and possibly occurring comorbidities have been considered purely static. In order to understand the causal relationships, however, a diathesis stress model is necessary, as has been customary in other areas for a long time.

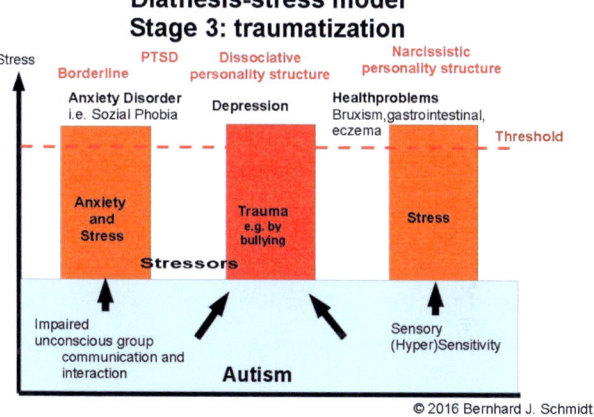

What is clear about this model is that autism, albeit still perceived differently, is NOT a disease. Autism is a version of human existence (neurodiversity) that was evolutionarily meaningful one or two centuries ago. The problems that often occur in autistic people arise depending on the socio-cultural environment and above all on anxiety and stress.

On the effects of stress on health e.g. by a negative influence on the immune system will not be discussed here.

Possible health problems as a result of anxiety and stress are:

   – **mental disorders such as depression, anxiety disorders, social phobia, ...**
      The occurrence of depression and concomitant suicidal tendencies should never be underestimated or overlooked!

"Persons with ASD but without intellectual impairment showed a higher mortality risk due to a specific cause: suicide.

'There is a very clear link between ASD without intellectual disability and a heightened risk of suicide,' said Drs. Hirvikoski. 'The clinical guidelines for suicidal patients must be strictly followed in people with ASD.'"

http://psylex.de/entwicklung/autismus/sterblichkeit.html

   – somatic diseases like
      - eczema,
      - gastrointestinal problems,
      - tooth damage,

- headache / migraine due to tension of the back / cervical muscles

- ...

These often occur in combination due to the same causes of anxiety and stress.

4 Further aftereffects

For the understanding of autistic people in the field of practice the knowledge about two further points is important:

4.1 „Intolerance of uncertainty"

Due to the lack of autopilot, that is, the lack of unconscious orientation to the group, autistic people always have to restructure their own world. This often leads to a strong intolerance against uncertainty. Because new, unexpected situations throw all plans and structures over the pile and can then easily lead to excessive demands in dealing with the respective situation.

4.2   „Insistence on sameness"

For the same reason, autistics often insist on equality, ie on the same processes and structures. In any case, the same structures and processes facilitate orientation and thus reduce anxiety and stress.

5   New perspective as a summary

Before switching to the practical part, here is a graphic summary of the different types of communication between NT people and autistic people:

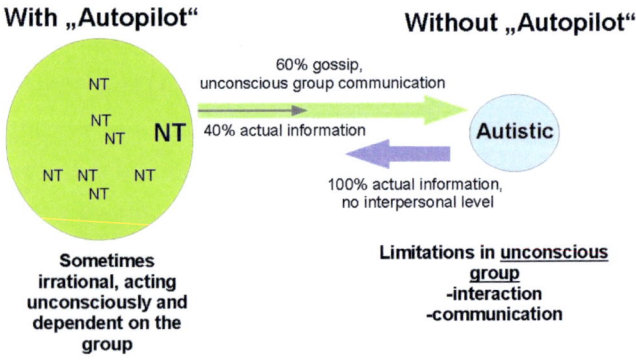

III. PRACTICE

The previously presented should have an impact on medical practice in three areas.

On the one hand, there is the effort to provide barrier-free access to practice for people in the autistic spectrum. For example, what has been guaranteed for years by suitable structural measures for people with physical disabilities must also be achieved in the near future by means of comparatively minor modifications of the practice organization, even for autistics.

Experiences with the reduction of mental barriers already exist in dental practices in dealing with anxiety patients. Awareness of both the problems of these patients and the need to remove barriers to make the visit to the doctor already exist here.

„In developed countries, around 5-15% of adults suffer from pathologically high dental anxiety, so they can only use dental help if they are in severe pain. About 3% completely avoid the visit to the dentist. Those affected suffer from severe dental sequelae and their psychosocial effects. Frequently, patients with phobia are recognized only after years of avoidance. Massive damage to the teeth are the result. Investigations on patients with a high

level of fear of dental treatment showed, in addition to the significantly poorer oral health, severe restrictions on oral health-related quality of life. Thomb et al. identified an average of eight teeth requiring treatment among dental phobics who had avoided visiting the dentist for many years. Many phobics are ashamed of the condition of their teeth and avoid speaking or laughing in public, and some withdraw from social life. The fear of visiting a dentist is so great that it can endure massive pain and postpone mandatory treatments. "

[Lenk M, Berth H, Joraschky P, Petrowski K, Weidner K, Hannig C: Fear of dental treatment—an underrecognized symptom in people with impaired mental health. Dtsch Arztebl Int 2013; 110(31–32): 517–22. DOI: 10.3238/arztebl.2013.0517]

At first glance, the problems of autistic people seem to be the same as those of anxiety patients. With the result that they often do not even appear in the doctor's office. But this impression is misleading, because the problems for Asperger autists are much more complex, they do not just refer to the treatment or the visit to the dentist. Although, of course, even in autistic people there may be additional treatment anxiety, but due to low pain perception treatment for autistic patients is often not the central problem, but rather the treatment environment. And not only at the dentist, but in all medical practices.

The second point is the consideration of the mentioned peculiarities in the anamnesis and diagnosis. This should affect in two directions. On the one hand, that diagnosed autistic patients increasingly ask about all stress-related illnesses. Often, these disorders occur together. On the other hand, in patients who do not have an autistic diagnosis but have the corresponding disease complex, autism should be considered as a possible cause, especially in older patients.

The third point in the treatment is the consideration of anxiety and stress as a cause necessary. Treatment of the indicated diseases in autistic people without a concomitant reduction of anxiety and stress can not be successful.

1   Accessibility

Unlike people who rely on a wheelchair, for example, accessibility for people with mental health problems requires essentially only minor changes in practice organization, as well as an understanding of the particular perceptions, behaviors, and specific types of communication of people in the autistic spectrum ,
In order to present these peculiarities, they are countered by questions from the HAF (Hierarchical Anxiety Questionnaire) by Prof. Jöhren to dentists.

21

Most important rule is, of course, due to anxiety and stress as main problems with Asperger autists,

avoiding anxiety and stress!

Even with the agreement and compliance with a doctor's appointment begin for many autistic people the problems!

– **Appointment**

Autistic people often have difficulties with telephoning. So here is the first hurdle for a practice visit. But this can be easily eliminated by

making appointments by email!

Autistic people are often overwhelmed with spontaneous communication over the telephone, so they make appointments that they can not comply with. Correcting or canceling these appointments, picking up the phone and calling the doctor's office means a lot of work. Make an appointment by e-mail, however, is stress-free.

– **Waiting room**

For autistics, the waiting room is a very special challenge.

The HAF question is: *"You are sitting in the waiting room, waiting to be called. How do you feel?"*

But the problem for autistic people is not waiting for the treatment, but the waiting room due to

1.) social phobia,

2.) hypersensitive olfactory perception and

3.) the "intolerance of uncertainty".

Because of the lack of "autopilot", ie the lack of unconscious group communication, as well as experienced exclusion and bullying, autistics often have a social phobia. Being close to other people in a room creates anxiety and stress.

Added to this is the olfactory perception of the body odors of other patients, especially in summer, which contributes to a pronounced malaise.

The uncertainty in the waiting room, when one is called and the treatment begins, leads to further stress. It follows:

The best is an appointment without waiting in the waiting room.

All this has nothing (as opposed to anxiety patients) to do with treatment as such. An appointment directly as the first patient in the morning or after the lunch break without waiting time serves to reduce anxiety and stress.

– **Treatment room**

Unfamiliar environments and changes are a major challenge for autistics. A familiar environment, on the other hand, provides security and helps reduce anxiety and stress.
Due to the "insistence on sameness" follows:

The best is always the same treatment room.

– **Reduction of sensory stimuli**

Certainly this is the point that is the hardest to implement. But the very knowledge that autistic people perceive their environment much more intensively and can not filter out disturbing stimuli is helpful.
The less sensory stimuli present in the practice, the less stress for the autistic patient. Here, too, autistics differ significantly from anxiety patients.
HAF question: "*Imagine you enter the treatment room and smell the typical **smell**.*"
and

HAF question: *"Imagine you **hear** the typical sound of the drill - how do you feel?"*
In autistic people the problem is not (alone) the connection between perception and treatment, as assumed in the HAF, but the perception due to hypersensitivity as such. So independent of a special treatment of a special field.

In addition to the perceived as unpleasant stimuli also include touches of the body, the skin. These should therefore be as little as possible and always be announced in advance.

2   Communication

As already stated, autistics communicate differently. This is of central importance both for the understanding of the autistic patient and to avoid misunderstandings as well as to be able to optimally carry out the treatment.

In autistic cases, the gossiping that is so pronounced in NT people, ie the "small talk", falls away. Autistic people do not unconsciously communicate about facial expressions, gestures etc.

It follows for the practice:

-     **no small talk**

While NT patients perceive small talk as positive and anxiety-reducing, it causes stress in autistic people. Well-intentioned gossip thus reaches the exact opposite in autistics.

In addition, it is difficult for autistics to filter out the relevant factual information from a diffuse mixture of small talk and factual information.

– Instead, clear communication of next action.

In order to avoid misunderstandings, to communicate information clearly and to reduce anxiety and stress in the autistic patient, a clear, relevant and continuous communication is necessary.

Using the example of questions from the HAF for anxiety patients, this is shown here:

HAF question: "*Together, look at the X-rays and **discuss** what to do.*"

HAF question: "*The dentist **tells** you that you have a tooth decay and that he wants to treat it now.*"

So a pertinent communication with the autistic patient about the upcoming steps, and not:

HAF question: "*He changes the position of the chair and prepares an injection.*"

For the autistic, the unpredictable and the unforeseen are the cause of anxiety and stress!

So the next actions should always be announced, especially if the autistic patient is touched.

3   History / Diagnosis

The consideration of anxiety and stress as the main problems of autistic and at the same time cause of many diseases is of central importance in the history and diagnosis. And this in two directions, depending on whether an autism diagnosis already exists or not.

3.1   In the case of existing autism diagnosis

If an autism diagnosis is made, all relevant diseases should be queried, regardless of the discipline! These are particular

1. Eczema
2. Gastrointestinal problems
3. Headache / Migraine
4. Back pain
5. Dental problems
6. Anxiety disorders

7. Social phobia

8. and in particular depression

9. ...

If necessary, the autistic patient should then be referred (together with the communication of the autism-specific treatment requirements) to appropriate specialists.

3.2 For several diseases from the anxiety / stress complex

Even older patients, who grew up at a time when autism was not yet conscious, have no diagnosis, but suffer from the corresponding diseases. A combination of neuro-dermatitis, social phobia / anxiety disorders and depression is not uncommon here.

For the treatment as well as the understanding of the causal relationships it is necessary to clarify whether the patient is from the autistic spectrum.

A diagnosis is carried out by specialized clinics.

4 Treatment

Of course, the treatment also has to take into account the reduction of anxiety and stress!

The pure treatment of the respective symptom without

simultaneous reduction of the causes, namely anxiety and stress, can not lead to success.

For example, without this reduction, you will not be able to do the dental care as fast as the patient is damaging his teeth by crunching. And that also during the day, which is why a bruxism track has only a limited effect.

For a long-term improvement of the "Health Related Quality of Life" attention to anxiety and stress as causes of diseases in autistic people and the detection of all acute diseases is necessary.

IV. EPILOGUE

Unfortunately, there is currently a big gap between the frequency and severity of health problems of autistic individuals on the one hand and their share of practice patients on the other hand.

So far, this has not only led to a severely limited health-related quality of life, but also to an increased risk of premature death.

The diseases involved in these problems can be found in almost all fields of medicine.

The elimination of the hurdles and barriers that are in the way of an adequate supply of people from the autistic spectrum, however, is achievable with manageable resources!

On the one hand, it is the understanding of autism-specific behavior and communication.

On the other hand, a slight modification or expansion of the practice organization.

If you have a proportion of autistic people in their practice that is proportionate to the population, then you can expect adequate care for those patients who are most frequently affected by illness.

V. BIBLIOGRAPHY

Schmidt, Bernhard J. (2015/1): Autistic and Society. An angry Change of Perspective. Vol. I: **Understanding Autism**. Norderstedt: Books on Demand.

Schmidt, Bernhard J. (2015/2): Autistic and Society. An angry Change of Perspective. Vol. II: **Support for Autistic**? Norderstedt: Books on Demand.

Schmidt, Bernhard J. (2016): Plaintext compact. **The Asperger Syndrome – Between Bullying and Inclusion**. Norderstedt: Books on Demand.

Schmidt, Bernhard J.; Ganz, Andreas (2016): Plaintext compact: **The Asperger Syndrome - not only for Psychotherapists.** Norderstedt: Books on Demand.

Schmidt, Bernhard J.; Döhler, Christiane and Deniz (2018): **Autism – Sexuality – Relationships.** Norderstedt: Books on Demand.

Schmidt, Bernhard J. (2019/1): **Autism and the Refrigerator Mother Myth. A Rehabilitation of Bruno Bettelheim.** Norderstedt: Books on Demand.

Schmidt, Bernhard J. (2019/2): Plaintext compact. **The Asperger Syndrome – for Parents.** Norderstedt: Books on Demand.

Schmidt, Bernhard J. (2019/3): Plaintext compact. **The Asperger Syndrome – for Teachers.** Norderstedt: Books on Demand.

Schmidt, Bernhard J. (2019/4): Plaintext compact. **The Asperger Syndrome – for School Assistants.** Norderstedt: Books on Demand.

Schmidt, Bernhard J. (2019/5): **Autism – Flight or Fight. New Perspectives on Challenging Behaviors.** Norderstedt: Books on Demand.